The Natural Cure for Erectile Dysfunction

How to Cure Erectile Dysfunction and Impotency Permanently in the Comfort of Your Own Home by Following These Simple and Easy Proven Methods

By Michael Cesar

Table of Contents

Introduction

For centuries, men have been associating their value as men with their jobs, their bank account, their physique, and their virility. Our contemporary culture has flooded our mind's eye with images of the "perfect man"—one who possesses the right job, the right family, and with a trip down to the local pharmacy, nights of virile intimacy.

But there are often consequences to the proverbial "happiness in a bottle."

This book will explore alternative and much healthier methods to deal with the sensitive issue of erectile dysfunction. It's time for men to realize that there is life beyond the pharmacy counter, beyond what our contemporary culture tells us is acceptable, and it's time to delve into centuries-old remedies that build up, not tear down our system.

I want to thank you and congratulate you for purchasing the book, *The Natural Cure for Erectile Dysfunction: How to Cure Erectile Dysfunction and Impotency Naturally in the*

Comfort of Your Own Home. By purchasing this, you're taking charge of your own physical and mental well-being as a man. You'll discover things like Ayurveda and the herb shilajit, and you won't be disappointed.

Thanks again for purchasing this book. I hope you enjoy it!

Chapter 1:
No Shame

Since the beginning of time, men and women have had expectations laid upon them, benchmarks that are established before even the first word is uttered. Men are supposed to be strong, caring, aggressive, and virile. Anything short of those in any way is considered to be insufficient and thus begins the psychological spiral into self-doubt. As we age, the messages and expectations become more concise and directly related to our sexual virility and performance.

To say that our contemporary culture is filled to overflowing with commercial messages about pharmaceuticals that will be the magic bullet and solve all of a man's problems in the bedroom is an understatement. Sporting events, news programming, and even prime time "family" television programs are sponsored by the likes of Cialis, Levitra, and Viagra. The depictions are of that of a happy middle-aged man with a more than attractive woman at his side, eagerly awaiting intimacy.

The opposite effect takes place, however, to men with any type of erectile dysfunction because the visual message is that unless steel-bending erections are normative, the viewer is less than a man—a man who has yet to fulfill his destiny. Well, the good news is that there are alternatives, so there need not be shame with these types of intimacy issues. As a matter of fact, the National Institutes of Health's studies show that as many as 5% of men aged 40 have this issue and 15–25% of men aged 65 suffer from erectile dysfunction on a long-term basis.

Erectile dysfunction has become a joke, a punchline for late-night comics and that fact alone only serves to add more weight to the stigma. Young children even poke fun at the attributes of the "little blue pill," and for men who suffer from erectile dysfunction, it's no laughing matter. It's unfortunate, but there are potential solutions that transcend pharmaceuticals, as you will find later.

The reasons for erectile dysfunction are many, ranging from a lack of stimulus from the brain to improperly functioning nerves in the penis to insufficient blood flow to the penis, to deeply felt and experienced emotional trauma, sexual incompatibility, and fear of intimacy.

There is also a school of thought that contends one contributing factor to sexual dysfunction is the over-accessibility of pornography. The unrealistic environments and circumstances portrayed in pornographic material hardly represents reality and the human mind becomes increasingly desensitized to normal, average sexual encounters. As the intensity of pornography increases, more is required to stimulate the viewer's mind. The shear pervasiveness of pornography is alarming enough, but the regular consumption therein reduces the ability to truly be connected with a partner in a physical, spiritual, and emotional manner.

Whatever the cause, the pharmaceutical answers aren't without side effects and introduces other health problems to the individual such as flu-like symptoms, nausea, headaches, and more. Whenever there is a disclaimer about seeking the aid of a physician if there is a problem, it should serve as a glowing area of concern.

In short, you're not alone and there is actually good news out there—there are treatments beyond shoving chemicals down your throat, and we're going to cover some of them shortly.

Chapter 2:
Mind and Body Effect on Erectile Dysfunction

When the mind and body aren't in sync, there are a myriad of problems that can and will eventually manifest themselves. Stress is but one example of the modern problems that permeate the fabric of the human existence and stress can, as the saying goes, kill. Stress can not only be a contributing factor to erectile dysfunction, but can lead to insomnia, colds, frequent infections, headaches, and a lack of energy. Combined, these symptoms and manifestations can destroy the contact between mind and body and result in difficulty in relaxing, avoidance of other people, and even low self-esteem.

As always, it's important to see a physician before any treatment regimen is launched to ensure there aren't deeper, more tragic health problems that could be the causal factors for erectile dysfunction.

For some men, there are psychological or emotional causes for erectile dysfunction, which creates a disconnection between mind and body. It could be sexual confidence, a traumatic experience, increased pressure at work, or even trouble in a current intimate relationship can be a contributing factor to that first incident of lack of function and then, the spiral can begin. The mental stress of being able to perform a sexual act becomes so overwhelming that an erection is elusive. Because there is a lack of sexual function, there is increased stress. Because there is increased stress, there is a lack of sexual function. And the cycle continues.

Now we begin the process into the mind through Tantra and how this intensely spiritual practice can change everything.

Chapter 3:
Tantra Cure for Erectile Dysfunction

Tantra is described as a belief or practice which believes that the universe in which we live in is a physical manifestation of divine energy that the godhead (higher power) uses to maintain the universe. Tantra seeks to channel that energy, to use that energy in the human experience, and to enhance the quality of life for the individual and the culture as a whole. It is an ancient practice dating back to the 5th century in Asia (some scholars date it as far back as 2000 B.C.) and the word "Tantra" itself is Sanskrit for "woven together"—to weave together the transcendent and the human experience. Tantra is not a religion but rather techniques designed to focus on spiritual enlightenment.

Tantra has been successfully used to overcome erectile dysfunction, and the process itself can be exciting as it introduces something new and challenging to both the physical and spiritual aspect of the human pathos.

This takes place in your very own home and not in a sterile, clinical environment. At home, there is no pressure and the mind is more open to receiving energy and stimulation.

The first thing that has to happen is an opening of the mind, a dismissal of preconceived notions of Tantra. You'll need to be open to exploring something completely different, perhaps something that seems totally strange and foreign to you initially. Some of the rituals, for example, may seem a little odd at first—such as the romantic rituals like the breathing techniques or the calming chants. Regardless of how uncomfortable you may feel at the beginning, dismiss that discomfort as a new door opening that you must enter. It's the start of a process to wholeness, to connectedness with the Tantra, and your partner.

The next step is introspection, an evaluation of self and priorities. It's a tough process, to be certain. No one really enjoys taking that inventory of both good and bad elements of our lives, but it is something that must be done. Fundamentally, everyone is different. The answers you seek and the solutions you desire are unique to you. The process of introspection, of personal inventory, is important because Tantra is wide-reaching, covering many concepts and encompasses thousands of years of tradition.

But first, let's develop some healthy meditation techniques.

Tantric Meditation

This can be done either alone or with a partner. In some cases, the stress of erectile dysfunction alone can contribute to erectile dysfunction; therefore the mind must be clear, open. Begin with locating a peaceful place with no distractions—no television, no smart phone, no Internet, no children, and no external noise. Get comfortable and begin breathing deeply and concentrate on how your stomach feels and how your diaphragm expands and contracts as you breathe. Take a deep breath and empty completely.

Try to use isometric exercises—the tightening and subsequent relaxing of each muscle group, beginning with your feet and working all the way up to the top of your head.

Traditional Tantric meditation is a reminder that those performing this form will have the goal of being conscious of the life force within each individual and the couple as a whole. In this, you begin by focusing attention at the base of the spine, traveling up to the neck and reaching its climax at the forehead.

After no less than thirty minutes of intense meditation, you will experience a sense of renewing, an awakening of new energies or a tapping into the energy that has been elusive.

Be Playful, Spontaneous, and Conscious

One of the most fundamentally important elements of Tantra is the belief that every human being possesses both the Shiva and Shakti (Tantric words for yin and yang)— both feminine and masculine aspects of their being. The man should feel free, comfortable to be vulnerable to his mate, and the processes of Tantra, when followed properly, will accomplish just that. It isn't about parading about in a dress or for the woman to wear a lumberjack's outfit, but rather about taking in and embracing the whole being of man and woman with no shame, no fear.

Discover Yourself

As you begin, you will take inventory of the messages your body is giving you—what you're smelling, what you're feeling, and what you're hearing—from the top of your head to the bottom of your feet. Mentally, start focusing on experiencing pleasure in the sexual experience, not the orgasm itself.

Do this when you are alone and when no one can disturb you. Make sure not to rush and do not forget to switch off your mobile phone, TV, etc. You can do this while standing, sitting, or lying down. Take off all your clothes and try not to be judgmental about your body, rather seeing beauty in yourself. Now begin slowly, from the top of your head and move downwards, going through your different body parts by gently touching, feeling, looking, hearing, and smelling—using all your five senses. Do not forget your private parts as they are import to be discovered again differently than you are normally used to. It is important to be playful, spontaneous, and conscious.

Discover Your Lover

Now it is time to discover your lover through Tantra and let your lover discover you. It is essential that both feel comfortable doing this together. Start simple with your lover by doing things together like breathing together, staring into one another's eyes deeply and tenderly. Attempt to take in one another's peace and energy. Now start to discover your lover's body by touching, feeling, smelling, tasting, and hearing—using all the senses. Your partner will remain conscious in body and opening up him/herself and being in the moment. When you both feel that it is time to shift, do so.

Next, you and your partner need to examine the totality of your physical and sexual needs and determine if they are compatible. Much has been written regarding sexual compatibility and some theories are painfully misleading. Keep in mind that it is not necessary that your goals be identical for Tantra to be effective, but when you have an understanding of what each other's needs are through Tantra, the stress of the sexual act itself is greatly diminished.

An integral part of this process is breathing. Often taken for granted, it is so crucial that in yoga a whole art form is dedicated to breathing called pranayama. It is what unites your body, mind, and even your consciousness, and it serves to help the Tantric practitioner maintain focus on the here and now.

Chapter 4:
Yoga Cure for Erectile Dysfunction

All men do not have a partner to practice yoga with and that's perfectly fine. The goal is the cure and the cure will open up many more relationship opportunities with confidence. Yoga will play a critical part in your cure for erectile dysfunction. The word itself means "to join together." As you can see, it cannot be divorced from Tantra. There are Hatha and Kundalini yoga techniques. Hatha is the yoga of the physical body and is ancient in its origin, whereas Kundalini yoga is a spiritual yoga with a focus on meditation and controlled breathing, resulting in energies necessary for sensuality.

One position for a man to do while alone is called Kandasana. Warm up first. Sit with your legs out to the front and bending the legs at the knees, bring the heels close to the perineum. Using your hands, place the soles of your feet against your navel—don't worry about slipping, you will do so on the first few tries but don't give up. Release your hands and press the palms against each other. Keeping your back erect, continue this pose for thirty minutes. Slowly and gently lower your legs to the floor. This activates muscles in the navel and stimulates sexual energies.

Next is a pose called Matsyasana which means "fish posture." This is most beneficial when done in the morning. Lie down on your back with legs straight, then bend the knee to try to make an arch, lifting the chest up and then raising the whole trunk. Push the floor with the elbows, the head backward resting on the crown. Forearms and arms will be used for support. After reaching this position, breathe deeply and slowly. As you release this pose, do so gently and with patience. This pose has been proven to be a great assistance in increasing sexual function.

Practicing the following poses with a partner will open up the experience, heighten the awareness and increase the psychological and spiritual aspects of the sexual act, spilling over into the physical itself. This is where the physical and spiritual meet and impact the efficacy of erections.

What are the benefits of yoga? Not only will the body be relaxed and strengthened, but the state of mind is improved. The physical positions of yoga are very similar to sexual positions, which makes for a perfect transition to sexual activity.

Here is where you begin with a partner:

Start by facing your partner. Put your hands together, palms touching and chant a simple chant such as, "Om Namah Shivaya." It is a primal chant, defining you as one who seeks a path of higher states of consciousness. Breathe calmly, concentrate on exuding love, peace, and harmony with your partner.

Happy Hug

Face each other with the tips of your toes touching and hug each other. Let yourself go in your partner's arms and take five deep breaths in unison. Take a deep, relaxing breath that fills you and slowly exhale and with it, release your tension, and your stress.

Tree Together

This position is begun by standing side-by-side with your partner. Wrap your arm around the waist of your partner, pick up your outside foot and bring it to the inside of your knee. Keep your legs strong and firm. Imagine they are roots in the ground and take several deep breaths and then switch positions with your partner and repeat.

Tantric Twist

With your backs touching, legs crossed, twist around to your left and place your left hand on your partner's right knee and place your own right hand on your left knee. Relax your neck, your face muscles while pulling on your partner's knee, take deep breaths simultaneously with your partner and then switch directions and repeat.

Lotus Pose

While all of the yoga positions are designed to be intensely spiritual and create connectedness with your partner, this pose is particularly spiritual. Sit cross-legged with feet resting on opposing thighs, facing each other. Ensure your knees are touching, join hands and let them rest between the two of you. Close your eyes and focus on the energy that is created between the two of your bodies and imagine you're intertwined. Focus on your partner's energy and lose yourself in each other's energy. This can go on as long as you like. Come out of the pose when you're both moved to do so.

These yoga exercises are to be done together with a partner and the gentle touching, the connectivity, spiritually, can begin to heal, to strengthen sexual arousal, and open the door for normative sexual function. The goal, remember, is to have the sense of togetherness, the weaving together of your consciousness with the divine and in so doing, to overcome erectile dysfunction.

The next aspect of the Tantra experience is the purpose and benefits of Pranayama breathing.

Chapter 5:
Pranayama Cure for Erectile Dysfunction

Pranayama is a Sanskrit word that means "lengthening of the life force." Prana (life force) flows through literally thousands of energy channels, centers called "chakras." The quality and quantity of the Prana determines one's state of mind and the mind is a significant element in erectile dysfunction. Regular practice of these Pranayama breathing techniques helps the Prana level be at a high and smooth, steady flow, resulting in a calm, relaxed mind.

To begin with Pranayama breathing, sit on a chair or on the floor with your legs crossed and your spine erect then take few deep breathes and relax your shoulders. Remember not to overdo and start gently and with fewer minutes. When you feel comfortable and can breathe more slowly, increase.

There are many Pranayama breathing techniques, and here are a few.

Bhastrika

The first is called the Bhastrika (Bellows Breath). Breathe deeply through the nostrils, feel the diaphragm moving, allowing the lungs to expand and gently force the abdomen out. Next, breathe slowly out through the nostrils—the process should be much slower than the process of inhaling. Continue this process for five minutes.

Kapalbhati

Another is called Kapalbhati (Shining Forehead). Breathe in deeply through the nostrils, deliberately. Forcefully exhale through your nostrils—you will feel the contraction of your stomach muscles. Repeat this for five to ten minutes, taking care not to hyperventilate. Always listen to your body and do not force yourself.

Anulom Vilom

Yet another is Anulom Vilom (Alternate Nostril Breath). Close your eyes and completely focus on your breathing. Close the right nostril with your right thumb and inhale through the left nostril. Fill the lungs with air, remove the thumb from your right nostril, keeping your hand close to your nose. Using the ring and middle finger, close your left nostril and breathe out slowly. Switch hands and repeat the process for up to ten minutes or less, listening to your body.

Chapter 6:
Tantric Massage Cure for All Sexual Issues

The purpose of Tantric massage is to receive kundalini energy (Kundalini: A potential force in the human existence, a residual power of pure desire and sensual energies.). It's a ritual of sorts and should be considered and dealt with as such. The massage itself adds energy and healing and the result is an awakening and nurturing of your sensuality. It creates an environment free of stress and makes your body feel fully alive.

Tantric massage can cure erectile dysfunction, impotency, premature ejaculation, inhibited ejaculation, sexual inexperience, and pornography addictions or sexual addiction as well as other sexual issues.

Self-Massage

Self-massage has been proven to be an excellent resource to cure erectile dysfunction. In the event that there is pressure, stigma, or self-consciousness because of the erectile dysfunction, performing massage as a couple may not be beneficial right away.

In Tantric terminology, the term "lingam" refers to the penis. That's where we begin, with self-lingam massage. The purpose here is not orgasm, therefore there is no pressure placed upon yourself. The purpose is heightened sexual self-awareness. Use a small amount of oil on the penis and testicles. Gently massage the oil onto the genitals, moving down to the perineum (found between the anus and testicles). Return to the shaft, taking your time, breathing deeply and intentionally, taking in all of the senses and energy being produced. There is what is called a "sacred spot" where you travel next. Between the testicles and the anus, there is a pea-sized spot. Delicately press inward and feel the pressure within. It may not be comfortable at first, but over time, the feelings become more and more intense.

When you're finished with the massage, it will be evident to you. Usually, these massages can last anywhere from five to thirty minutes, keeping in mind the goal of sexual awareness and that awareness will eliminate erectile dysfunction.

Couple's Massage

The role of the receiver in the couple's massage is to stay present in the moment, to feel and absorb every touch being made and to take deep, soothing breaths—in through the nose, out through the mouth—and it helps you to stay in that very moment and move the sensual kundalini through your whole body.

The role of the giver in Tantric massage is simple: To touch in a way that feels good to the giver. That's right, the giver. You see, if there is touch that feels good to us as we give, it will feel more fulfilling to our partner and it is the partner's erectile dysfunction that will be cured. In addition, it forces us to think about the enjoyment of being the giver and how it is feeling to the recipient. It makes the giver get out of his/her head for a few moments and truly consider the enjoyment of the recipient as well.

To begin, have the recipient lay on his/her belly and remember as the giver, the most important element is to touch lightly, slowly. It may feel uncomfortable at first as the giver usually isn't used to this type of massage. Focus on the touch itself, using deep breaths in pace with the recipient.

Explore the whole body as if it were completely new to you. Follow where the massage leads, move wherever the giver chooses. This is a full body massage, so don't forget the whole body. The back massage will end when it needs to, when the timing feels right and when it happens, the recipient should roll over. Begin this next phase of the massage slowly, hands on the chest of the recipient, breathing together slowly, passionately, and deliberately.

Gender is irrelevant as to who is receiving the massage, as the whole body is to be massaged including sensual zones. The kundalini will rise and fall as these sensual areas are touched and awakened, and that is perfectly fine. Don't try to control the happening—it is doing what it is supposed to. The ritual, that is, the Tantric massage, will end at its own time and when it does, the focus should be on breathing, taking in the deep levels of relaxation. It's a caring, loving ritual designed to increase connectedness, and the end result will be less stress and decreased incidents of erectile dysfunction. You will begin to awaken the divine energy within you.

The misconception about Tantra massage is the "happy ending" myths—it is designed to produce more than one orgasm by relaxing mind, body, and spirit and taking focus away from the actual act of orgasm itself. The sexual organs are often included in a Tantric massage, but it is to celebrate the sensuality, not the release of bodily fluids as an end to a means. As a matter of fact, Tantric massage is designed to produce more than one orgasm and those are to be deeper, more intense.

Far too often, people tend to think of the sexual organs as distant, as cut off from the rest of the body and spirit therefore it is difficult to avoid dysfunction unless the whole being is included in any sensual act. Tantric massage can and will produce an orgasm, but it is not at all to be considered mere masturbation. To look at it that way is tantamount to looking at prayer as a little more than a short nap.

As an integral part of the Tantra, you'll next see what benefits Ayurveda, holistic systems of healing as a part of the cure for erectile dysfunction, brings to the experience and how all aspects work together to help your body, mind, and spirit. When those are whole, erectile dysfunction becomes a thing of the past.

Chapter 7:
Ayurveda Cure for Erectile Dysfunction

Ayurveda is one of the oldest holistic systems of healing both the body and the mind known to man. The goal is to prevent illness, and millions of people today live healthy and well-balanced lives because of it. If the body begins to develop diseases, Ayurveda can provide the right remedy to each individual in the attempts to cure and bring the body back to its natural balance. Ayurveda is important to sustain balance in body, mind, and consciousness through diet, regular exercise, relaxation, a consistent cleanse, and meditation.

Ayurveda is close to 5,000 years old and is part of the overall correction and treatment of erectile dysfunction.

Vajikarana: To Be Like a Horse

The treatment of erectile dysfunction is called Vajikarana therapy in Ayurveda. Vajikarana is one of the eight branches of Ayurveda. This type of therapy increases the strength and virility of a man to perform sexual acts—to be like a horse, as it were. Vajikarana is truly comprised of three basic elements:

- A disciplined lifestyle.
- Conditional sex act based on the assumption that sex is not only for pleasure.
- The use of Vajikarana aphrodisiac medical formulations.

This discipline is focused on increasing will power and holding the Shukra (semen) for a longer time. Vajikarana deals with sexuality as a whole, addressing the anatomy, physiology, pathology, diet, and medicines (aphrodisiacs) involved in sex.

Each of these elements are not designed to be isolated from another or dissected to not be a sum total of its working parts. The massage, the meditation, the yoga, and the supplements work together in unity during the Ayurveda experience to cure erectile dysfunction. It's spiritual as well as mental and physical, and it is so to ensure connectivity between the body, the mind, and the divine power.

In the next chapter, we'll cover some of the herbal remedies that have been found to be effective in treating erectile dysfunction and sexual dysfunction as a whole.

Chapter 8:
The Healing Power of Diet and Herbs

Ayurveda/Ayurvedic physicians or therapists combine herbal formulas, diet changes, exercise, and relaxation techniques (thus the meditation discussed in Chapter 3) to help men overcome sexual dysfunction through safe and natural means rather than be dependent upon pharmaceutical chemicals. Vajikarana therapies has led to good strength, increased happiness, longer spans of erections, and heightened potency.

Diet

In our contemporary culture, it's difficult to avoid unhealthy foods filled to overflowing with chemicals and additives as well as food that is made from animal proteins. These proteins contain bacteria and hydrochloric acid at such a rate as to be dangerously unhealthy. It's important to note, however, that following the pathways of Ayurveda does not mean that everyone must absolutely follow a vegetarian diet. And it may not be wise if the body has disease or allergies to foods.

Fresh fruits and vegetables including: cereals and grains, fruits containing high concentrations of seeds, citrus fruits, apples, melons, peaches, celery, and green leafy vegetables reduce risk of illnesses that have been known to cause erectile dysfunction such as diabetes and liver disease, among others.

In essence, avoiding foods that have long been touted as having a negative impact on health is an important part of effective Tantra. Fried foods, fatty foods, sugary foods, and the like can all have a negative impact on the body and thereby create a fertile environment for disorders that contribute to sexual dysfunction as well as erectile dysfunction.

It's time to review a few of the Ayurvedic and other herbs that are available and have helped in eliminating erectile dysfunction.

Shilajit

Also known as the "Indian Viagra," shilajit has many useful benefits such as keeping calcium in the bones and thereby making them stronger. It serves as an anti-inflammatory, an antioxidant, and a memory enhancer. The most important benefit, however, for the purpose of this book is improving male sexual function. It has also been used for centuries to increase libido itself—a significant contributing factor to erectile dysfunction.

Some of the properties of shilajit are beneficial for people suffering from: anemia, bronchitis, hemorrhoids, kidney stones, diabetes, arthritis, asthma, thyroid dysfunction, and even obesity. It is also known to be an aid to those desirous of increased physical performance over all. It improves natural strength gain and reduces down time post workout.

If used properly and in tandem with proper diet and exercise, shilajit is not known to have any severe side effects. If you're taking exceedingly high doses however, it might increase a uric acid level which, in turn, becomes problematic for bile levels. Increased bile levels can impact the gallbladder and the liver alike, leading to acute digestive problems. As always, it's important to discuss this and other supplements for erectile dysfunction with a physician before taking any supplements whatsoever.

Ashwagandha

This herb is an aphrodisiac for men by stimulating the natural production of nitric oxide in the body. Nitric oxide opens up the blood vessels carrying blood to the genitals. It's recommended to take 2 grams of Ashwagandha in the evening and though it may take a few days of consistent usage to see results, an opening of blood flow to the genitals is important to curing erectile dysfunction.

Gokshura

This herbal supplement increases the secretion of testosterone and thereby has the properties of an aphrodisiac. It's been known to cause sexual arousal in both men and women. Gokshura also increases the blood flow to the genital area by enlarging and opening up blood vessels. Effects usually take place after three days of continued usage when taken in 1–3 gram doses.

Maca

Maca is a plant in the broccoli family and the roots resemble turnips a great deal. Maca has been used as an aphrodisiac traditionally and has been used to aid both genders. In men, it's been reported to have increased the libido as well as sperm production. Fortunately, it does not work through hormones therefore there will be no increase of testosterone—only natural biological reactions to plant material used for increasing libido.

Maca has also been reported to increase energy, stamina and reportedly, enhance mental clarity. In human studies, it has been known to increase the volume of semen in ejaculation for men, and for women, it may assist with menstrual problems and hormonal imbalances.

Ginseng

If you have familiarity with Chinese medicine, you'll recognize this herb. There are typically three types of ginseng—Asian, Siberian, and American. Ginseng is a centuries-old remedy for sexual function primarily because it works on the reproductive and nervous systems to increase libido. By working on the blood vessels in the penis, it helps to improve erections. It is available in an extract, powder, a paste, or you can get it in capsule form. If you choose a concentrated extract, 100–200 milligrams should suffice. Ginseng may take a few days to produce results and it's important to note that individuals with heart or kidney problems or even high blood pressure should talk to their physician about ginseng.

L-arginine

L-arginine is, at its core, an amino acid that increases the amount of nitric oxide levels in the human body. Nitric oxide is a substance, a molecule, that tells "smooth muscle" to relax and, as a result, the blood vessels dilate and increases blood flow (essential for maintaining erections).

L-arginine can be found in foods such as chicken, fish, peas, and walnuts as well.

Combined with a healthy commitment to the Tantra and effective diet and exercise, these techniques studied here will greatly help in the reduction of instances of erectile dysfunction.

> Note: Always check with your physician prior to taking any herbs or supplements.

Chapter 9:
Healthy Tips to Combat Erectile Dysfunction

Erectile dysfunction has become a common complaint from men in our contemporary society, and many have reached out to the centuries-old methods of Ayurveda. We've covered the Tantra that includes breathing techniques, yoga, relaxation, and meditation and then considered diet and natural supplements.

Now, we take a walk down the enlightened path of common sense, and remind ourselves of some very good, very healthy tips that can rectify erectile dysfunction.

Avoid alcohol. Alcohol directly impacts the central nervous system and can cause erectile dysfunction. Excessive alcohol consumption can also lead to debilitating diseases such as cirrhosis that also causes erectile dysfunction.

Do not be afraid. As we discussed in a previous chapter, the fear of not being able to perform sexually can lead into a spiral of disappointment and endless fear. Use the techniques given freely in this book to eliminate fear and build confidence.

Exercise will keep the cardiovascular system healthy and studies have proven that men who exercise regularly have fewer problems with erectile dysfunction. And exercise makes you feel better and perhaps live longer.

Sleep. A body that has experienced high-quality rest is more energized. Rest is an essential element to human survival.

Just say no. Heroin, cocaine, marijuana, and other illegal drugs will most assuredly cause erectile dysfunction eventually and are horribly dangerous and hazardous to the body.

Masturbation. Reduce the frequency of masturbation to no more than twice a week. Tantric massage is never to be confused with masturbation.

Body massage. Massaging the whole body with herbal oils once a week increases sexual energy and stamina. Body massage is one of the best and most effective aphrodisiacs in Ayurveda.

Lose the extra poundage. Losing weight helps to increase testosterone levels as well as sexual energy and stamina. Obesity will lead to hypertension and diabetes. Diabetes can cause erectile dysfunction, and the medications necessary to keep hypertension under control also cause erectile dysfunction.

Psychotherapy. Anxiety associated with sexual performance and sexual activity can be minimized with healthy psychotherapy. Working together with a partner willing to help with development of intimacy will aid in relieving anxiety and thereby reducing the instances of erectile dysfunction.

Increase your libido! Lacking libido is often regarded as a woman's problem, but men can also suffer from a low sex drive resulting in erectile dysfunction. In addition to the herbal supplements mentioned previously, increasing zinc, vitamins A, C, and E, and using ginseng can help with sex drive also!

Hit a workshop. Tantra workshops are available locally, most often where yoga is practiced. The face-to-face interaction of fellow sojourners in the Tantra experience will provide a unique insight you can't get anywhere else. As mentioned in Chapter 1, you're not alone.

Togetherness. Include your partner in every part of the Tantra, get them involved in the process and don't be shy to openly discuss these problems and issues. It will benefit both partners greatly.

Detox. Cleanse the body from toxins at home. Buy from an organic shop or search the Internet for a good product that is safe and mild to use at home.

Panchakarma which is an Ayurvedic detox cleanse, vitalizes the body, and along with Vajikarana therapy, can be done at an Ayurvedic clinic.

Stop smoking or intake of all forms of tobacco if you are suffering from ED.

Never forget that this is a process of enlightenment of the mind as well as the body—an awakening to the divine nature, the essence of the creation itself. Tapping into the energies of Tantra improves not only the sexual urges and performance, but makes for a better human being.

Conclusion

Thank you again for purchasing this book! By doing so, you've joined a group of men and women who desire more from life, who want to live life to the fullest, and to solve a serious problem that is more intense than just a few commercials make it seem.

I hope this book was able to help you to learn about the possibilities of healing and of improving your sensual existence through the participation in Tantra.

The next step is to live. Be happy. Share what you've learned with your partner and with those within your sphere of influence. This transcends mere "hippie talk," but sensitively addresses the proverbial "elephant in the room" with a divine essence. The goal is unity, connection. Not alienation.

Finally, if you enjoyed this book, then I'd like to ask you for a favor. Would you be kind enough to leave a review for this book on Amazon? It'd be greatly appreciated!

Thank you and good luck!

Glossary of Terms

Tantra: Tantra is described as a belief or practice which believes that the universe in which we live is a physical manifestation of divine energy that the godhead (higher power) uses to maintain the universe.

Yoga: Yoga is a physical, emotional, and spiritual practice with the goal of transforming the body and mind to have connectedness.

Kundalini: A potential force in the human existence; a residual power of pure desire and sensual energies.

Meditation: A practice where the user trains the mind to both concentrate intensely and let go freely. Used to focus energies and open the mind, body, and spirit to connectedness.

Ayurveda: Has 8 components (Curing of disease, treatment of children, surgery techniques, cure of specific diseases of the E.N.T., deals with causes that are invisible such as spirits, antidotes for poisons, rejuvenation, healthy sensuality and procreation). Ayurveda is one of the oldest holistic systems of healing both the body and the mind known to man. Its goal is to prevent illness, and millions of people today live healthy and well-balanced lives because of it.

Other books by Michael Cesar:

Tantric Sex—The Sacred Union Of Souls
Improve Your Sex Life And Your Relationship with
Tantra

The union of two people on more than a physical level is the ultimate goal as you read through this book. Once you allow yourself to be one with your partner and the divine, you will experience true sexual freedom and lose your inhibitions with your partner.

The Natural Cure for Erectile Dysfunction
How to Cure Erectile Dysfunction And Impotency
Permanently In The Comfort of your own Home By
Following These Simple And Easy Proven Methods

Discover how to finally overcome Erectile Dysfunction, impotency, premature ejaculation, inhibited ejaculation, sexual inexperience, pornography addictions, or sexual addiction as well as other sexual issues.

Success Habits
Kaizen — Improve Your Life and Become Successful by Taking One Small Step at a Time

This book is a dynamic resource for men and women alike to set small, attainable goals that are measurable and maintain a pattern of positive behavior. "Kaizen" means "change for better," and is created to increase your productivity at work as well as at home.

Ayurveda Weight Loss
The Ultimate Guide to Successful Ayurvedic Detox and Weight Loss

This book covers the cleansing/detoxification process, the Ayurvedic diet, the lifestyle changes, as well as tips and aids for daily life and maintaining commitment to your weight loss goals and personal goals.

Effortless Manifestation Magic And Miracles
Discover The Single Most Powerful Method Of Manifesting Your Dream Life From Oneness

Within the universe lays a wealth of information that the human mind has only just begun to tap into. Manifesting is one of those sources which are readily available to anyone who seeks to obtain the miracles that the universe is waiting to impart on every individual. Similar to prayer and meditation, manifesting is a personal journey into the magic of self-discovery and a unique oneness with the world around us.